The Road to Successful CRT Implantation

A step-by-step approach

The Road to Successful CRT Implantation

A step-by-step approach

Daniel Gras MD

Interventional Cardiology Care Unit
Nouvelles Cliniques Nantaises
Nantes, France

Angel R. León MD, FACC

Chief, Cardiology
The Linton and June Bishop Chair of Medicine
Associate Professor of Medicine
Emory University
Atlanta, GA

Westby G. Fisher MD, FACC

Director, Cardiac Electrophysiology
Evanston Northwestern Healthcare
Assistant Professor of Medicine
Feinberg School of Medicine
Northwestern University
Evanston, IL

Foreword by

William T. Abraham MD, FACC

Professor of Medicine
Chief, Division of Cardiology
The Ohio State University
Columbus, OH

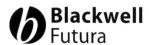

© 2004 D. Gras, A.R. León and W.G. Fisher
Published by Blackwell Futura, an imprint of Blackwell Publishing

Blackwell Publishing, Inc., 350 Main Street, Malden, Massachusetts 02148-5018, USA
Blackwell Publishing Ltd, 9600 Garsington Road, Oxford OX4 2DQ, UK
Blackwell Science Asia Pty Ltd, 550 Swanston Street, Carlton, Victoria 3053, Australia

First published 2004

ISBN: 1-4051-1718-4

Catalogue records for this title are available from the British Library and the Library of Congress

Acquisitions: Gina Almond
Production: Tom Fryer
Set in Sabon by Sparks

For further information on Blackwell Publishing, visit our website:
www.blackwellfutura.com

The publisher's policy is to use permanent paper from mills that operate a sustainable forestry policy, and which has been manufactured from pulp processed using acid-free and elementary chlorine-free practices. Furthermore, the publisher ensures that the text paper and cover board used have met acceptable environmental accreditation standards.

Notice: The indications and dosages of all drugs in this book have been recommended in the medical literature and conform to the practices of the general community. The medications described do not necessarily have specific approval by the Food and Drug Administration for use in the diseases and dosages for which they are recommended. The package insert for each drug should be consulted for use and dosage as approved by the FDA. Because standards for usage change, it is advisable to keep abreast of revised recommendations, particularly those concerning new drugs.

Contents

Dedication, vii

Foreword, ix

General remarks, 1

1 How does ventricular dyssynchrony alter hemodynamic function?, 4

2 What clinical benefits can we expect from CRT?, 6

3 How to select candidates for CRT, 8

4 Assessment of ventricular dyssynchrony by new echocardiographic analyses, 10

5 What are the mechanisms of improvement during CRT?, 12

6 Clinical situations where CRT is unlikely to be of therapeutic value, 14

7 Preimplantation checklist, 16

8 Right versus left-sided approach to implant the CRT system, 18

9 Right ventricular pacing in CRT, 20

10 How to achieve reliable sensing and pacing of the right atrium, 22

11 Is it safe to pace the left ventricle via a coronary sinus tributary?, 24

12 Why perform a coronary sinus venogram before placement of the left ventricular lead?, 26

13 Optimal LV lead positioning, 30

14 How to manage difficult coronary sinus cannulation, 32

15 How to avoid a dissection of the coronary sinus ostium, 36

16 How to overcome a myocardial bridge over the coronary sinus, 38

17 What to do in the absence of a lateral branch on the venogram, 40

18 How to manage high left ventricular pacing thresholds, 42

19 How to proceed in the presence of a complex coronary sinus anatomy, 44

20 How to manage diminutive target coronary sinus tributaries, 46

21 What to do when valves are in the way, 48

22 How to implant a CRT system in the presence of a left superior vena cava, 52

23 Dilatation of the target cardiac vein by angioplasty techniques, 56

24 Stenting for recurrent dislodgment of the left ventricular lead, 58

25 Assessment of the electrical signal sensed by the left ventricular lead, 60

26 How to avoid stimulating the left phrenic nerve, 62

27 Dye extravasation and venous perforation or dissection, 64

28 How to avoid a cardiac vein dissection by the balloon catheter, 66

29 How to remove the guiding sheath using the slitting technique, 68

30 Radiographic appearance of the final lead position of the CRT system, 70

31 How to implant a CRT device in patients with chronic atrial fibrillation, 72

32 Upgrading DDD pacing to CRT, 74

33 Upgrading a CRT to a CRT-ICD system, 76

34 Repositioning of a dislodged left ventricular lead, 78

35 How to implant a four-chamber CRT system, 82

36 How to implant a biventricular, double-left ventricular lead CRT system, 84

37 Alternatives in left ventricular lead implant failures, 86

38 Left ventricular lead extraction, 88

39 Management of ventricular double counting in CRT, 90

40 Management of non-responders to CRT, 92

References, 95

Index, 97

Dedication

To my wife and the kids; for their continuous understanding, infinite patience, and love.

To all of those who, step by step, contributed to the development of CRT.

To the patients who participated in key studies on CRT, so others could further benefit from this new treatment.

Foreword

Heart failure is a major and growing public health problem, affecting more than 22 million people worldwide. Despite effective drug therapies, heart failure morbidity and mortality remain unacceptably high. Cardiac resynchronization therapy (CRT) represents a new approach to heart failure management. Results from numerous observational and randomized controlled trials have consistently demonstrated significant improvements in quality of life, functional status, and exercise capacity in NYHA class III and IV heart failure patients assigned to active resynchronization therapy. In these patients, cardiac resynchronization has also been shown to improve cardiac structure and function, while significantly reducing the risk of worsening heart failure. Preliminary results from another large-scale trial have suggested a significant reduction in all-cause mortality as well as the combined end-point of all-cause mortality and all-cause hospitalization with cardiac resynchronization therapy in an advanced heart failure population. Thus, cardiac resynchronization therapy not only makes heart failure patients feel better, it also helps them to live longer.

In 2001, the first resynchronization device became commercially available in the United States. The next year, two devices that combine biventricular pacing capability with implantable cardioverter defibrillators (ICDs) were approved for use by the U.S. Food and Drug Administration. Recently updated *ACC/AHA/NASPE Pacemaker and ICD Guidelines* included cardiac resynchronization therapy as a Class IIA recommendation for pacing. Patients with ischemic or nonischemic dilated cardiomyopathy, interventricular conduction delays, and New York Heart Association class III or IV symptoms are currently candidates for CRT.

The device is implanted in the sub-pectoral region in a similar manner to a conventional pacemaker or ICD, with placement of three electrodes to pace the right atrium and each ventricle. Pacing the left ventricle requires accessing a cardiac vein in a dilated, disease-deformed heart that belies our knowledge of gross anatomy. As with any new procedure, skills are built by repetition and the sharing of experience. This book is recommended both for physicians currently implanting CRT systems, and those in training. It is organized by 40 questions developed from 10 years of experience in developing this new procedure, and training hundreds of new implanters. The authors' combined experience of more than 3000 procedures provides a means of flattening the learning curve with a wide variety of clinical examples. Their experience may help direct you through the difficult procedures, thus permitting the application of this valuable therapy to all eligible heart failure patients. The overwhelming change in patient lives that can occur with CRT is not possible without the skills of the device-implanting physician.

William T. Abraham MD

General remarks

The key contributions of long-term cardiac resynchronization therapy (CRT) as a supplemental treatment of refractory congestive heart failure have recently been reported. Several completed studies support the validity of this new therapy, which improves left ventricular (LV) and mitral valve function, quality of life and exercise capacity, and decreases the need for hospitalizations. These gains, however, hinge not only on a careful patient selection but also on a proper lead placement, particularly the lead responsible for LV stimulation.

The implantation of a CRT system may now be achieved without major difficulties in 80–90% of patients, thanks to recent advances in technology dedicated to the LV lead placement. Unexpected obstacles may, however, be in the way of an uncomplicated procedure in approximately 10–20% of cases. This may have serious consequences since an improper LV lead placement is a source of unsuspected procedural failure, where, despite effective capture of all stimulated cardiac chambers, no clinical improvement is observed from lack of resynchronization.

Whether the LV lead is best inserted from the right or left subclavian approach remains unsettled. The right-sided approach allows an optimal fluoroscopic visualization of posterior or lateral cardiac veins in a left anterior oblique (LAO) projection without conflict between fluoroscopic equipment and surgical exposure. This consideration is not relevant when a defibrillating system is included since active pulse generators are best implanted in the left pectoral region.

In early CRT system implants, the LV lead was introduced first, such that, if that failed and there was no indication for conventional cardiac pacing, the procedure was terminated. This practice has now been mostly abandoned, after the relatively frequent observation of traumatic right bundle branch block (RBBB) during attempts to catheterize the coronary sinus (CS) with the guiding sheath, resulting in complete heart block and, occasionally, prolonged ventricular standstill, forcing the rapid implantation of a right ventricular (RV) lead at a site that may have been less than optimal. The current high success rates of LV lead placement allow the fixation of the RV lead, usually in the mid-septal region, as a first procedural step. In the rare cases where the LV lead implantation procedure fails, an alternative may be to implant a CRT device connected to the right-sided leads and proceed with an epicardial approach for LV stimulation.

1

Implantation of the LV lead is the critical phase of the procedure, and should be preceded by angiographic visualization of the CS and its tributaries, in search of the optimal implantation site. The ultimate choice of a vein for LV stimulation will depend on the highly variable anatomy of the coronary venous system. The aim is to place the myocardial lead in a lateral tributary of the CS, in order to stimulate a late-activated region and coordinate LV segmental contraction. In the absence of a lateral vein, or when it is tortuous or at an excessively sharp angle to the CS, other vessels may be accessible, including the posterior vein, which normally originates shortly past the CS ostium. Alternatively, an antero-lateral vein originating from the great cardiac vein, or a mid-cardiac vein, may allow access to a posterior region around the LV apex. These various lead positions may be indistinct on antero-posterior (AP) fluoroscopy, and must be verified in the LAO projection.

Since this therapeutic approach is recent, it is important to be familiar with the procedure-related complications that have been identified thus far. First, complications encountered with conventional cardiac pacing may be more common with CRT. A subclavian venous puncture is currently indispensable to introduce the guiding catheter needed for CS angiography and placement of the LV lead, increasing the risk of pneumothorax when compared to the cephalic approach, which may be preferred for traditional right atrial (RA) and RV leads implantation. Furthermore, the overall duration of a CRT system implantation is longer than that of a conventional DDD pacemaker, involving several added procedural steps mostly devoted to positioning of the LV lead. This, in particular, may increase the risk of infectious complications, mandating the enforcement of especially rigorous sterile techniques. Second, a difficult cannulation of the CS may cause traumatic RBBB, usually resulting in complete atrio-ventricular (AV) block of unpredictable duration in this population of patients with preexistent left bundle branch block (LBBB). Implanting the RV lead first may prevent this. Third, though they have become less frequent with the use of new, perfected, soft tip guiding catheter, perforation or dissection may occur during CS catheterization. In most cases, it is uncomplicated, and the implant procedure can be completed. In rare cases, the development of pericardial effusion and tamponade may require emergent therapeutic measures, including pericardiocentesis. Fourth, left phrenic nerve stimulation can be prevented by meticulous testing of the LV capture threshold at the time of system implantation. This may force the choice of another LV stimulation site, and limit the benefits expected from CRT. New pulse generators with independent RV and LV channels allow finer adjustments of the LV output voltage, and mostly eliminate phrenic nerve stimulation.

Instrumentation dedicated to the implantation of CRT systems has been developed to facilitate the placement of the LV lead and minimize the risk of serious complications, which, in our experience, occur in less than 1% of procedures. The advice, directives, and maneuvers described in this monograph are based on actual procedures. They intend to assist medical personnel involved in the implantation of CRT systems, with a view to facilitate the learning process, optimize practical applications of the techniques, prevent or overcome complications, and bring this procedure to a level of complexity comparable to the implantation of DDD pacing systems.

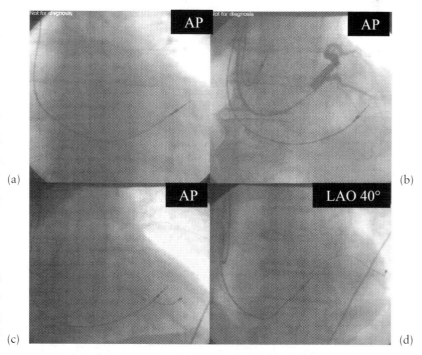

(a) (b) (c) (d)

Typical CRT implantation. (a) RV lead is implanted first, by the active fixation of a bipolar electrode to the mid-interventricular septum. (b) RA lead is then implanted, by the active fixation of a bipolar electrode to a site able to provide reliable sensing and pacing. (b) CS angiography is performed to identify cardiac veins of interest for chronic LV pacing. (c) An over-the-wire LV lead is implanted in a lateral vein. (d) LAO 40°. Final RV and LV lead positioning is better evaluated by using a LAO projection.

1 How does ventricular dyssynchrony alter hemodynamic function?

Cardiac dyssynchrony describes the loss of homogeneous segmental LV contraction. This abnormality of mechanical LV contraction is due to delays in impulse conduction through the diseased myocardium, which often develop during the evolution of ischemic and non-ischemic dilated cardiomyopathy. The pathophysiology of ventricular dilatation causes local conduction abnormalities, usually predominant in the distal ramifications of the Purkinje network and manifest on the surface electrocardiogram as left axis deviation of the QRS or LBBB. The associated delay in ventricular activation further decreases the LV ejection fraction (EF), and increases intracavitary pressures and wall tension (Fig. 1a). The delayed contraction of the postero-lateral LV wall and lateral papillary muscle promotes functional mitral regurgitation by preventing the proper coaptation of the valve leaflets. The delay and prolongation of LV contraction also shortens the diastolic filling period, which, in the late phase of the disorder, may overlap the late atrial filling period. This latter phenomenon may be accentuated by prolongation of the PR interval and acceleration of the resting heart rate. In addition, abnormal LV filling may decrease coronary perfusion (Fig. 1b).

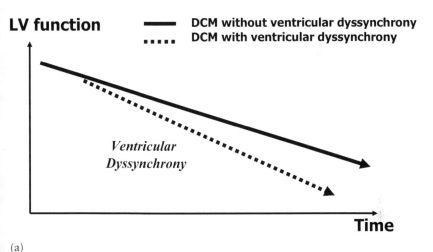

(a)

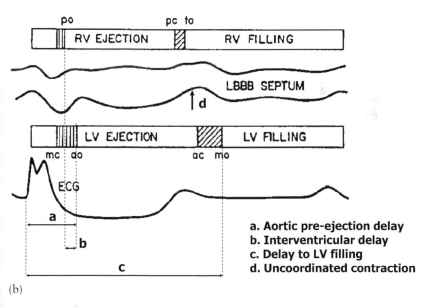

(b)

Fig. 1 (a) LV function, showing DCM without ventricular dyssynchrony and DCM with ventricular dyssynchrony. (b) Interventricular septal motion in left bundle branch block (LBBB) and the relation to dynamic ventricular dyssynchrony. DCM, dilated cardiomyopathy. Reproduced from Grines *et al*, *Circulation* 1989; **79**: 845–53, with permission from Lippincott Williams & Wilkins.[1]

2 *What clinical benefits can we expect from CRT?*

Several multicenter studies have confirmed the efficacy of CRT, which has now been added to the armamentarium available to manage chronic congestive heart failure (Fig. 2). The results have been both concordant and remarkable, including a significant decrease in New York Heart Association (NYHA) functional class, increase in exercise capacity measured by 6-minute hall walk or maximum oxygen consumption, and improvement in quality of life. These clinical benefits are associated with an increase in LVEF, an improvement in LV filling function and, over the long term, reverse LV remodeling. Additional benefits include a decrease in the number and duration of hospitalizations, whether due to cardiac decompensation or not. The impact on survival has not been formally established, though seems highly likely, in view of the results of a meta-analysis,[2] and of the outcome of the COMPANION trial prematurely interrupted by the Data Safety Monitoring Board.[3] The CARE-HF trial, which closed its patient enrollment in March 2003, should contribute complementary information regarding the impact of CRT on survival.[4]

	Study	Patients	NYHA Class	QoL Score	Hospitali-zations	6 Minute Walk Test	Peak VO_2	LV Size/ Function
	French Pilot [5]	50	+	na	na	na	+	na
	InSync (Europe, Canada) [6,7]	103	+	+	na	+	na	+
	InSync ICD (Europe) [8]	84	+	+	na	+	na	na
RANDOMIZED TRIALS	MUSTIC [9,10]	58	na	+	+	+	+	+
	PATH CHF [11,12]	41	+	+	+	+	+	+
	MUSTIC AF [13]	43	na	↔	+	+	+	na
	MIRACLE [14,15]	453	+	+	+	+	+	+
	PATH CHF II [16]	89	+	+	na	+	+	na
	MIRACLE ICD [17]	369	+	+	↔	↔	+	↔
	Contak CD (Class III/IV) [18]	227	+	+	↔	+	+	+
	MIRACLE ICD II [19]	186	+	↔	↔	↔	↔	+
	Contak CD (Class II) [18]	263	↔	↔	↔	↔	↔	+
	COMPANION [20]	1520	na	na	+	na	na	na

Key. + = CRT favorable; ↔ = CRT neutral; na = not available or reported

Fig. 2 Summary of the results showing the efficacy of CRT.[5–20]

3 How to select candidates for CRT

Cardiac resynchronization is currently a therapeutic option for patients in NYHA functional class III or IV, who have a dilated cardiomyopathy refractory to optimal medical therapy and dyssynchrony of ventricular mechanical function. Dilated cardiomyopathy is defined as an LVEF ≤ 35% and an LV end-diastolic diameter ≥ 55 mm. Optimal medical therapy includes diuretics, angiotensin-converting enzyme inhibitors, and, if tolerated, beta-adrenergic blockers and spironolactone.

Ventricular dyssynchrony is of foremost importance, since it is the element of the disease that CRT intends to rectify. It is apparent as a QRS complex duration ≥ 130 ms or, perhaps more importantly, on the basis of echocardiographic criteria developed to confirm that intraventricular conduction abnormalities correspond to dyssynchrony of contraction and relaxation. As an example, the selection criteria applied in the CARE-HF trial were (a) an aortic pre-ejection delay ≥ 140 ms (Fig. 3a), (b) an interventricular mechanical delay ≥ 40 ms (Fig. 3a,b), and/or (c) evidence of 'postsystolic contraction', or overlap of systole and diastole (Fig. 3c). The time between the onset of the QRS to the beginning of aortic ejection (Fig. 3a) is significantly delayed after the pulmonary ejection (Fig. 3b), which results in an interventricular mechanical delay of 110 ms.

Fig. 3 (a) Q to pulmonary ejection = 120 ms, (b) Q to aortic ejection = 230 ms, (a) and (b) prolonged aortic pre-ejection delay > 140 ms, interventricular mechanical delay = 110 ms, (c) postsystolic LV segmental contraction (LV postero-lateral wall).

- Dilated Cardiomyopathy: EF ≤ 35%, EDD ≥ 55 mm
- NYHA functional class III / IV
- Optimal medical treatment: ACEI, diuretics, BB, spironolactone
- Ventricular dyssynchrony
    - QRS ≥ 130 ms
    - QRS < 130 ms: CARE HF echo criteria (2 of 3)
        1. Aortic pre-ejection delay ≥ 140 ms
        2. Interventricular mechanical delay ≥ 40 ms
        3. LV segmental post systolic contraction

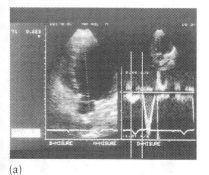

(a)

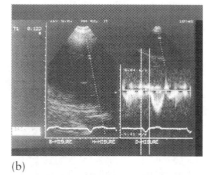

(b)

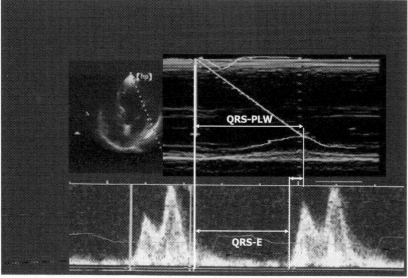

(c)

4 Assessment of ventricular dyssynchrony by new echocardiographic analyses

Tissue Doppler echocardiography is particularly helpful to identify the presence of ventricular dyssynchrony in patients whose QRS complex duration is < 130 ms. It allows a precise quantification of LV segmental contraction inhomogeneity and degree of mitral regurgitation. The most commonly measured variable is the left intraventricular delay, the interval between septal and posterior wall contraction.

Fig. 4 (a) Upper left panel: tissue Doppler image in the apical four-chamber view of a normal subject. Right panel: the velocity profile during one cardiac cycle obtained at the base of the interventricular septum. The solid lines mark the duration of systole (310 ms), and the arrow indicates the peak systolic velocity (8 cm s^{-1}). The diastolic filling of the LV is reflected in the E-wave (E) and A-wave (A). Lower left panel: tissue tracking displays, in color-coded format, the regional myocardial shortening (mm) in each segment, calculated automatically as the integral of the digitally stored velocity tracing in systole in each segment.
(b) One sample (A) is positioned at the base of the septum and another (B) is located in the posterior wall. In each point, strain rate (SR) analysis is carried out in a range of 10 mm. The first solid line (right panel) represents the onset of a negative SR in the septum (A line), indicating the onset of systolic shortening. The second solid line indicates cessation of systole, where the SR in the septum becomes positive. At the same time, a negative SR is observed in the posterior wall (B line), and this persists between the second and third lines, documenting shortening in early diastole (i.e., delayed longitudinal contraction).
Reprinted from Søgaard *et al.*, *J Am Coll Cardiol* 2002; **40**(4): 723–30, with permission from American College of Cardiology Foundation.[21]

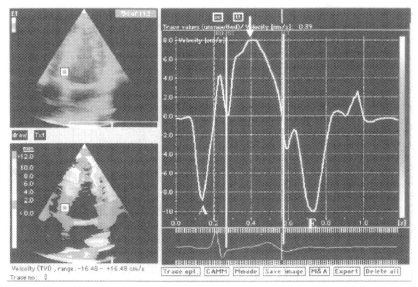

(a)

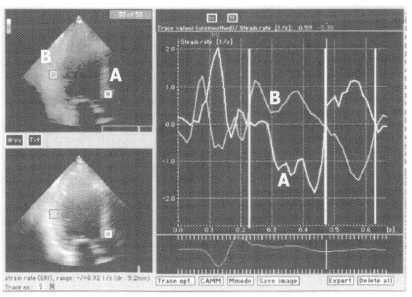

(b)

5 What are the mechanisms of improvement during CRT?

CRT improves LV systolic function by coordinating segmental contraction, resulting in an increase in LVEF. It is noteworthy that this improvement in LV systolic function takes place without increase in myocardial oxygen consumption, as opposed to the effects of inotropic drugs (Fig. 5a). Ventricular filling is also optimized by an increase in the filling period, along with a more physiologic transmitral flow pattern, i.e. a sharper separation between E and A waves. In several instances, functional mitral regurgitation is decreased as a result of a more synchronized postero-lateral wall LV contraction (Fig. 5b). Furthermore, long-term reversal of LV remodeling has been observed, suggesting that it may reverse the natural progression of the myopathic disorder. Finally, in preliminary studies, these effects have been associated with a positive impact on neuro-hormonal activity and indexes of heart rate variability.

Immediate

- LV function indexes
- LV filling phase
- Myocardial oxygen consumption
- Decrease in mitral regurgitation
- LV reverse remodeling effect

Delayed

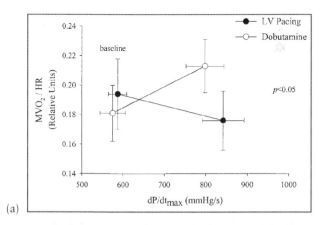

(a)

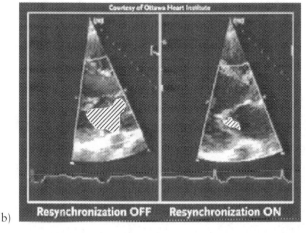

(b)

Fig. 5 (a) CRT improves LV function and decreases myocardial oxygen consumption. (b) CRT decreases dynamic mitral regurgitation. (Courtesy of Ottawa Heart Institute.) Reproduced from Nelson *et al.*, *Circulation* 2000; **102**: 3053–9, with permission from Lippincott Williams & Wilkins. [22]

6 Clinical situations where CRT is unlikely to be of therapeutic value

- Unstable coronary artery disease.
- Severe mitral regurgitation due to structural abnormalities of the valve apparatus.
- Severe aortic stenosis.
- Advanced RV dysfunction due to chronic lung disease or to end-stage dilated cardiomyopathy.

MUSTIC [10]

- Hypertrophic or restrictive cardiomyopathy
- Suspected acute myocarditis
- Correctable valvulopathy
- Acute coronary syndrome lasting less than three months
- Recent coronary revascularization (during the previous three months) or scheduled revascularization
- Treatment-resistant hypertension
- Severe obstructive lung disease
- Inability to walk
- Reduced life expectancy not associated with cardiovascular disease (less than one year)
- Indication for the implantation of a cardioverter–defibrillator

(a)

MIRACLE [23]

- Baseline 6-minute hall walk distance more than 450 meters
- Unstable angina, acute myocardial infarction, coronary artery revascularization surgery, or coronary angioplasty within the past 3 months
- Dependence on frequent intermittent (defined as more than 2 outpatient infusions per week) or continuous inotropic drug therapy
- Presence of pacing systems or indications or contraindications for standard cardiac pacing
- Severe primary pulmonary disease
- An existing implantable cardioverter defibrillator (ICD) or indications for an ICD, including those patients with sustained ventricular tachycardia (VT) within the previous month
- Chronic atrial arrhythmias (or cardioversion from such an arrhythmia within the previous month) or a paroxysmal atrial event within the previous month
- Supine systolic blood pressure of less than 80 mm Hg or more than 170 mm Hg
- Cerebral vascular event within the previous 3 months
- Cardiac allograph (patients on heart transplant list for the first time are not excluded)
- Enrollment in any concurrent study that may confound the results of this study
- Primary severe uncorrected valvular heart disease
- Supine resting heart rate of more than 140 bpm
- Serum creatinine more than 3.0 mg/dL
- Serum hepatic function 3 times the upper limit of normal
- Patients who are not expected to survive for 6 months of study participation because of other medical conditions
- Women who are pregnant or of child-bearing potential and who are not on a reliable form of birth control

(b)

Fig. 6 Exclusion criteria of primary CRT trials. (a) MUSTIC,[10] (b) MIRACLE.[23]

7 Preimplantation checklist

The following instrumentation should be readily available at the time of implantation of a CRT system:
- fluoroscopic equipment capable of capture and recall of images
- subclavian introducer sized for the guiding catheter sheath
- preferably a non-ionic contrast agent and means to administer
- various pre-shaped guiding catheter sheaths for CS catheterization (Fig. 7a,b)
- balloon catheter for CS angiography
- JR4 or multipurpose coronary angiographic catheter to facilitate access to the CS, if necessary
- long J and various 0.014 inch angioplasty guide wires
- electrical recording system to examine the timing of the ventricular electrogram with respect to the QRS complex on surface electrocardiogram.

In recipients of a previously implanted pacing system, the permeability of the subclavian vein needs to be ascertained.

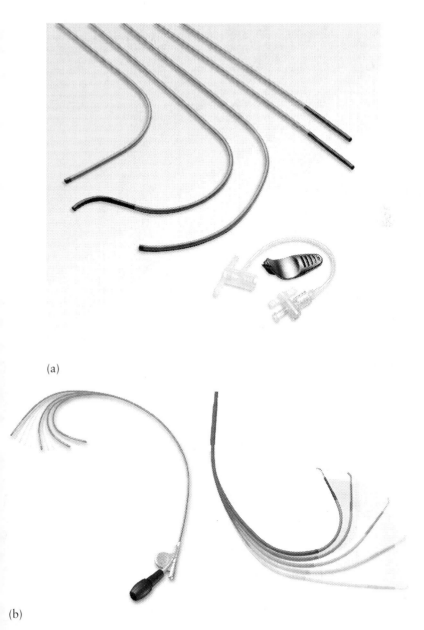

(a)

(b)

Fig. 7 Various catheters with different shapes to adapt to variant CS anatomy.

8 Right versus left-sided approach to implant the CRT system

Whether the LV lead should be implanted from the left versus right subclavian vein remains an open debate. In general, this choice depends primarily on the operator's practice and the layout of the laboratory. The right-sided approach facilitates fluoroscopy in the LAO projection and visualization of a posterior or lateral cardiac vein, without conflict between the imaging equipment and the operator (Fig. 8a). Advocates of a left-sided approach as a first choice generally recommend working in a sitting position to resolve this conflict. If the CRT device to be implanted includes cardioversion/defibrillation functions, the left side is preferred, since the average defibrillation energy requirements are lower when the active can is implanted in the left subclavian area (Fig. 8b). However, many recipients of CRT systems implanted on the right side have undergone upgrades to CRT-ICD with safe margins of defibrillation threshold. It is noteworthy that patients who underwent unsuccessful placement of the LV lead from the right subclavian vein had successful implantations from the left, and vice-versa. Therefore, operators should be familiar and comfortable with both approaches.

Fluoro Views

LAO   ### RAO

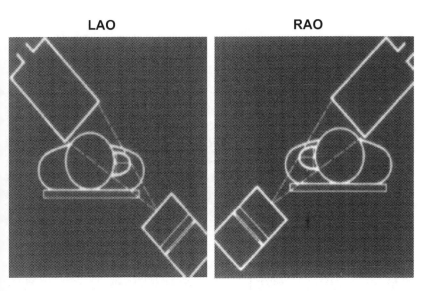

Subclavian vein occlusion:
Contralateral LV lead implantation

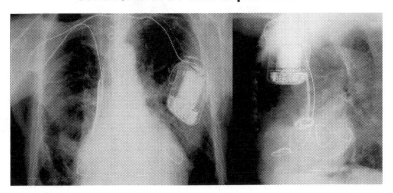

Fig. 8 (a) Right- versus left-sided approach to implant the CRT system. (b) CRT-ICD device implanted on the left while LV lead implanted from the right subclavian vein.

9 Right ventricular pacing in CRT

In the early CRT implantation experience, the LV lead was implanted first. If that failed, the procedure was terminated, unless there was an indication for conventional cardiac pacing. This practice was abandoned after the observation, during attempts to catheterize the CS, of traumatic RBBB in up to 20% of cases, resulting in complete heart block, sometimes without ventricular escape rhythm. Therefore, with the >95% success rate in LV lead implantation achievable currently, the RV lead is now implanted first.

The optimal site of RV stimulation remains uncertain, and most likely depends on the location of the LV lead. It also remains to be determined whether a subset of patients with severe RV dilatation and systolic dysfunction would benefit from RV stimulation at two separate sites.

At this time, RV stimulation is best achieved by the active fixation of a bipolar electrode into the mid-interventricular septum (Fig. 9a,b). This site avoids the known adverse hemodynamic effects of RV apical stimulation. In addition, it corrects for the septal contraction delay usually observed with LV stimulation, which, itself, intends to eliminate the delay of lateral wall contraction observed during spontaneous rhythm.

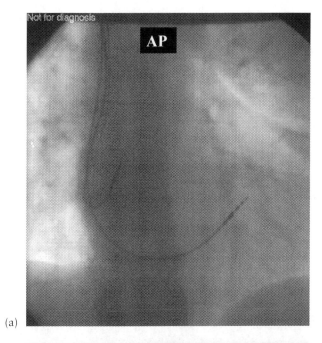

(a)

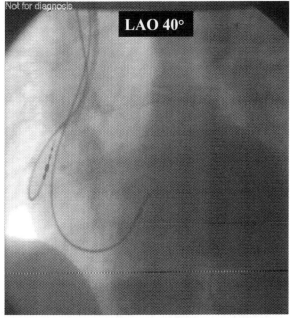

(b)

Fig. 9 RV lead positioned at mid-interventricular septum.

10 How to achieve reliable sensing and pacing of the right atrium

The atrial lead plays an important role, since it is responsible for the flawless preservation of atrio-biventricular synchrony, a central component of CRT. In these patients, the system usually operates in an atrial sensing mode, which implies the choice of a site associated with a high-quality RA endocardial electrogram. Implantation of the RA lead in the high lateral wall, near the sinus node, shortens the electro-mechanical delay, allowing earlier sensing of atrial activation, which may facilitate the subsequent programming of an optimal AV delay. On the other hand, one may consider, in patients with a history of paroxysmal atrial fibrillation (AF), to choose an atrial lead implantation site near the CS, with a view to decrease the incidence of arrhythmic events. Ultimately, in absence of firmly established rules, the optimal site is chosen on a case-by-case basis, and dictated by reliable sensing and pacing, preferably from an actively fixed bipolar lead (Fig. 10).

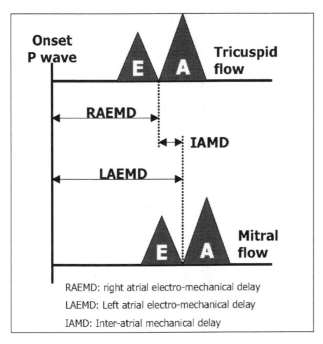

Fig. 10 Evaluation of right and left atrial electromechanical delays by using Doppler echocardiography.

11 Is it safe to pace the left ventricle via a coronary sinus tributary?

Permanent LV stimulation by a lead placed in a cardiac vein is not known to be associated with particular risks. The initial concerns of CS thrombosis have been dispelled by the absence of its report in a now abundant body of clinical experience. One should remember that, in the early developments of cardiac pacing, the atrial lead was implanted in the CS, since instrumentation available then did not allow its reliable placement within the RA cavity. The safety of long-term atrial pacing from the CS or from one of its tributaries was later reconfirmed with left atrial (LA) pacing performed for antiarrhythmic purpose and, more recently, with CRT.

Mechanical occlusion of a small cardiac vein and development of local fibrosis may occur, particularly when the lead body diameter is near that of the vein. The rich anastomotic network of the cardiac venous circulation makes this clinically inconsequential. Perforation of the CS or its tributaries may occur at the time of system implantation, but has not been reported during long-term follow-up. In large clinical trials, LV stimulation has generally been achieved with a mean capture threshold higher than typically observed in right-sided cavities, though has remained stable on the long term.

BIV Pacing Trials	MIRACLE	InSync III	Contak CD	MIRACLE ICD	Total
Implants attempted	591	334	517	636	2078
Implant success	92%	95%	87%	88%	90%
Procedural death	0.3%	0.3%	0.4%	0.4%	0.3%
30 day mortality	1.8%	1.8%	2.3%	1.0%	1.7%
LV lead complications	9.5%	4.0%	9.0%	12.0%	9.0%
CS trauma/complications	1%	1%	2%	4%	2%
Infections	1.0%	0.6%	1.6%	2.0%	1.3%

	PHD	1 month	3 month	6 month	12 month
Threshold @ 0.5 ms (V)	1.3±1.1	1.3±1.0	1.4±1.1	1.4±1.1	1.5±1.1
Impedance (Ohm)	747±195	695±166	732±180	737±174	767±185

Fig. 11 (a) BIV pacing trials.[24] (b) Data from the InSync III study for patients implanted with Attain® OTW Model 4193 (Medtronic, Inc.).[25]

12 Why perform a coronary sinus venogram before placement of the left ventricular lead?

CS angiography is a key step of the LV lead implantation procedure. It allows the visualization of target veins likely to achieve effective cardiac resynchronization, and those less suitable for placement of the lead. It also facilitates the anticipation of technical difficulties due to small venous diameters, sharp angles between target vein and CS, presence of valves, or tortuosities (Fig. 12b,c). These findings help choosing an appropriate pre-shaped lead and/or guiding catheter. The venogram is best performed at the time of LV lead implantation in order to take advantage of the support offered by the guiding sheath, which has become indispensable for the introduction of small (4F) over-the-wire leads.

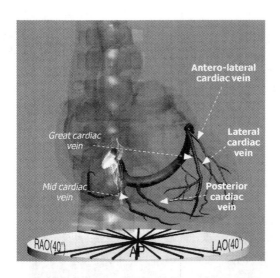

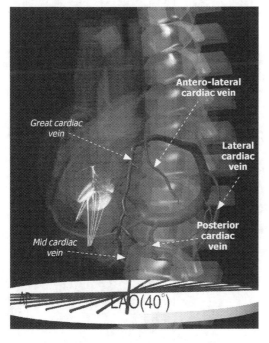

Fig. 12 (a) Coronary sinus venous anatomy. (*Continued.*)

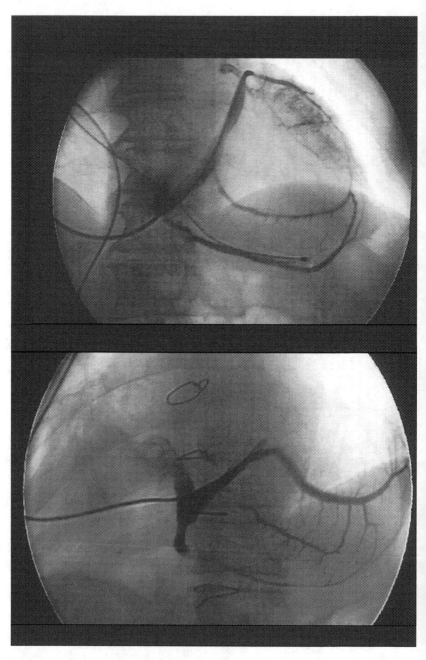

Fig. 12 (*Continued.*) (b) CS anatomy is highly variant.

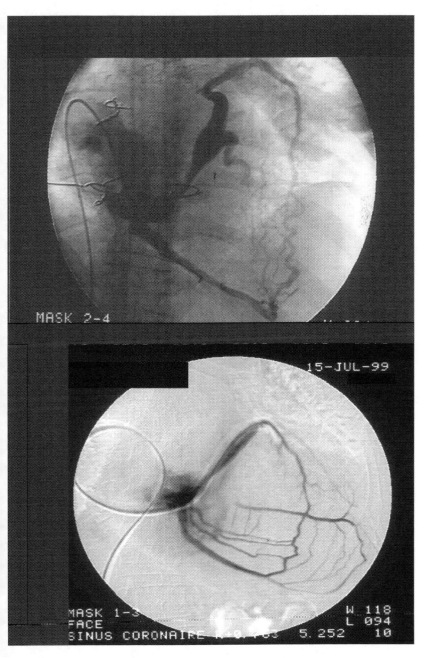

Fig. 12 (Continued.) (c) CS anatomy is highly variant.

13 Optimal LV lead positioning

Several multicenter studies have confirmed the postero-lateral wall as the site of LV stimulation associated with the best short- and long-term hemo-dynamic and clinical results. Conversely, stimulation of the LV apex or anterior wall is discouraged, since it is likely to have no or adverse mechanical effects, and may increase the amount of preexistent mitral regurgitation.

The LV lead should be placed in a lateral or posterior vein, or one of their branches, or, as a last resort, in an antero-lateral vein (Fig. 13). The great or middle cardiac veins, straddling the interventricular septum, should be avoided, as well as veins on the anterior and apical aspect of the LV, unless they are connected with anastomoses wide enough to reach the postero-lateral wall. The identification of these veins and of their course is best explored by multiple fluoroscopic views. The 30–60° LAO projection usually allows distinguishing of the various vessels that drain the posterior versus anterior territories, and avoids confusion between the middle and the posterior cardiac veins, or the great cardiac and the antero-lateral veins, which may be superimposed in the AP projection.

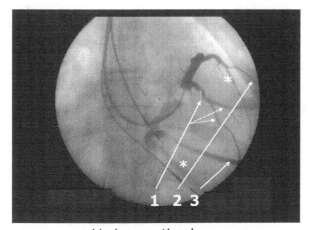

**Various optimal
LV pacing sites**
1.Lateral vein
2.Anterior lateral vein
3.Posterior vein

*** Non optimal LV
pacing site**
- Great cardiac vein
- Middle cardiac vein

Fig. 13 Identification of various LV pacing sites.

14 How to manage difficult coronary sinus cannulation

Several factors may hamper the catheterization of the CS, which must be identified during the procedure in order to adapt the choice of instrumentation. The more dilated the RA, the more difficult the CS access. The curvature of the guiding catheter may have to be widened, which may be accomplished by choosing a model adapted to the underlying atrial shape and size, or by using a dual catheter approach. The latter consists of introducing another 4 or 5 Fr JR4 (Fig. 14a, arrow) or multipurpose catheter, or a variable-curve electrode catheter to modify the distal curvature of the guiding sheath and facilitate entry into the CS.

A prominent Eustachian valve may prolapse in front of the CS ostium and hinder its catheterization. Choosing a hook-shaped guiding sheath or, in particularly difficult cases, the advancement of an electrode catheter via the femoral approach, will usually overcome this obstacle. A prominent Thebesian valve may also obstruct the proximal CS. The guiding sheath should be positioned at the ostium, to provide support, albeit precarious, and introduce an angioplasty guide wire, which should easily cross the valve. An over-the-wire LV lead can then be advanced directly, or a 4 or 5 Fr guiding sheath may be used as a brace to advance the lead to the mid CS. Another option consists of temporarily catheterizing the CS with an electrode catheter from the right femoral venous approach (Fig. 14b, single arrow), which serves to localize the CS orientation and facilitate the introduction of the guiding sheath from the superior approach (Fig. 14c, double arrow).

Changes in the geometry of the ventricles can cause a marked displacement of the CS ostium, which may become 'nowhere to be found'. As a last resort, an injection of contrast material in the left coronary artery and recording of the venous phase may help in localizing the CS ostium.

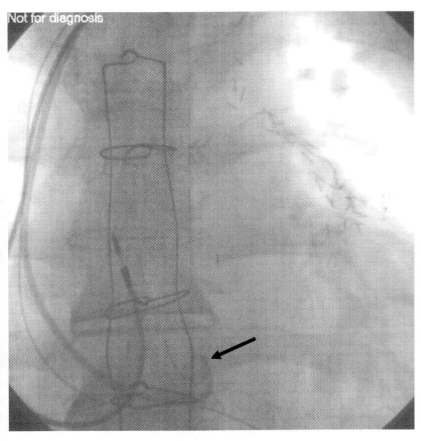

Fig. 14 (a) JR4 catheter introduced into guiding sheath to facilitate CS cannulation. (*Continued.*)

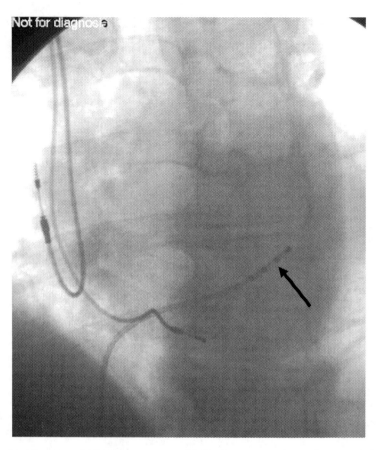

Fig. 14 (*Continued.*) (b) Management of difficult access to the CS due to a Thebesian valve.

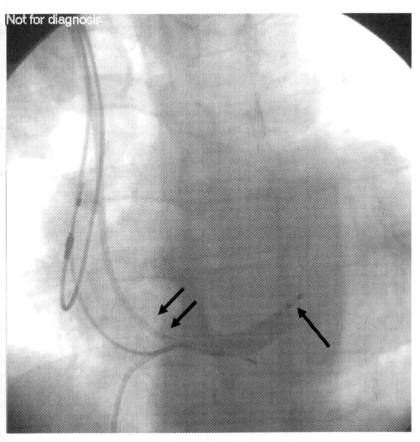

Fig. 14 (Continued.) (c) Usefulness of EP catheter introduced via femoral vein, to further cannulate CS ostium.

15 How to avoid a dissection of the coronary sinus ostium

Introduction of the guiding sheath may cause a dissection of the proximal floor of the CS. This complication, which occurs in <1% of cases, may have serious consequences, including tamponade, and is more likely with a rigid guiding sheath, when positioned perpendicular to the CS long axis (for example with an Amplatz catheter introduced from the right subclavian vein), or when manipulated forcefully. It can be easily avoided by observing the following steps:

1 visualization of the CS ostium by an injection of contrast material;
2 immobilization of the guiding sheath in front of the ostium;
3 introduction of a J guide wire, advanced far into the great cardiac vein (Fig. 15a,c);
4 catheterization of the mid CS by a 'push-pull' maneuver;
5 confirmation by another injection of contrast material of the proper placement of the guiding sheath within the CS, and not inside a tributary (Fig. 15b,d).

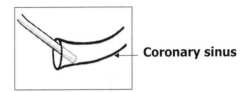

Coronary sinus

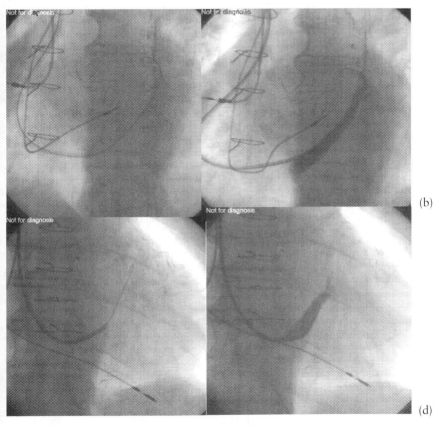

(b)

(d)

Fig. 15 CS cannulation using a 'push-pull' approach.

16 How to overcome a myocardial bridge over the coronary sinus

As observed over the coronary arterial system, myocardial bridges may course over the veins, particularly along the length of the CS. This can be suspected when, during a test injection of contrast material, the CS is narrowed or completely occluded during ventricular systole (Fig. 16a,b). If the venous compression is prominent, the use of a balloon catheter is discouraged, as it may injure the CS at the site of inflation. Instead, a venogram with 10 cm³ of contrast material is performed directly through the guiding sheath, which usually provides images of high enough quality to allow the selection of a target vein.

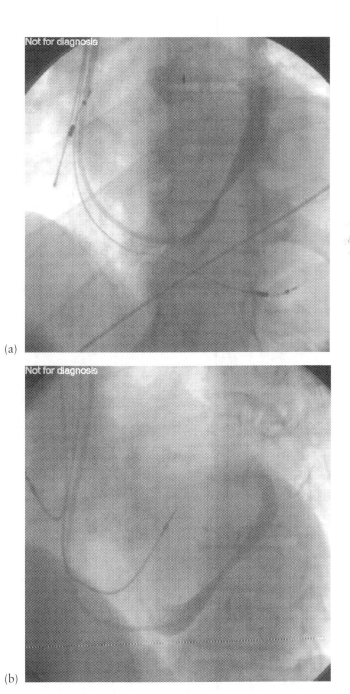

(a)

(b)

Fig. 16 Myocardial bridge over the CS.

17 What to do in the absence of a lateral branch on the venogram

The absence of an angiographically visible lateral cardiac vein denies the operator access to the optimal site of LV stimulation. To verify that the balloon has not been inflated at the very point of entrance of the vein into the CS, thus preventing its opacification, a second venogram should be performed after reinflation of the balloon in the proximal CS (Fig. 17a–c). If the lateral vein remains invisible, a large posterior vein with an ostium separate from that of the CS may be found and catheterized directly with the guiding sheath (Fig. 17d,e).

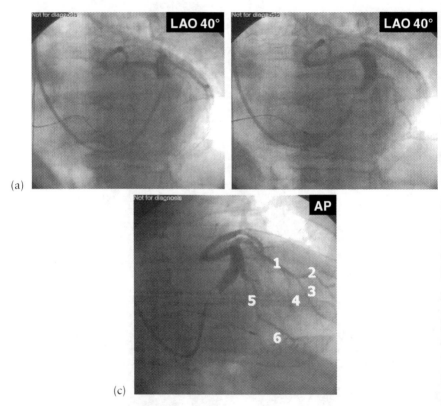

Fig. 17 (a,b) 1 vs 2 lateral veins after dye injection. (c) AV, showing six different LV pacing sites. (*Continued.*)

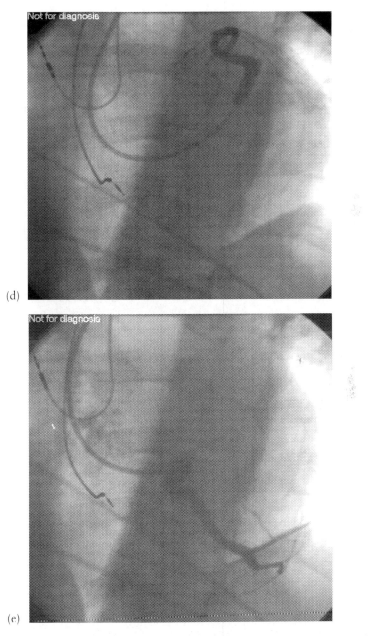

(d)

(e)

Fig. 17 (Continued.) (d,e) Posterior vein dominant when lateral veins are small.

18 How to manage high left ventricular pacing thresholds

The LV capture threshold is high when the electrode is near scarred myocardial tissue (Fig. 18a,b), or when abundant fat separates the vessel wall from the epicardium. A thorough exploratory venogram to establish a hierarchy of potential target veins is particularly important. When the lead has been placed in the target vein, alternate positions in nearby branches, or an altogether different vein draining a late-contracting territory, should be explored. In any case, it is noteworthy that the ultimate goal is not to obtain a low capture threshold, as is usually possible in a great cardiac vein (Fig. 18c), but to achieve effective resynchronization (Fig. 18d). Capture thresholds up to 4 V/0.5 ms may have to be accepted, at the cost of a shorter battery life, as long as the final system configuration improves ventricular function.

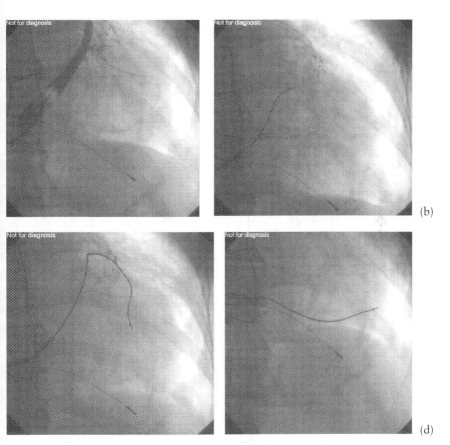

(b)

(d)

Fig. 18 (a,b) Appropriate LV lead location but high pacing threshold. (c) Good LV pacing threshold but inappropriate LV lead location. (d) Good LV lead location and good LV pacing threshold.

19 How to proceed in the presence of a complex coronary sinus anatomy

The target vessel may be difficult to catheterize because of tortuosity and/or sharp angulation at its entrance into the CS. Choosing an over-the-wire LV lead design facilitates the catheterization. Two techniques are suggested.

1 With the guiding sheath in stable position inside the proximal to mid-CS (1–2 cm below the target vessel entrance), the pre-shaped curve of the LV lead is used to cannulate the vessel up to the point of resistance within the tortuous segment. A coronary angioplasty guide wire of intermediate stiffness is advanced through the lead body and further through the tortuosity, as far as possible into the target vessel. If necessary, softer or stiffer guide wires may be exchanged. A pull (the wire) and push (the LV lead) maneuver is then applied to advance the LV lead, while keeping the guiding sheath in a fixed position (Fig. 19a,b).

2 If the pre-shaped LV lead curve cannot be introduced into the target vein entrance, the lead is replaced by a 4 or 5 Fr, JR4 or multipurpose coronary angiographic catheter, to cannulate the target vein, up to the point of tortuous resistance. The wire is then advanced, as described earlier, through the angiographic catheter, which is then removed to allow the over-the-wire LV lead placement into its target position. Larger-size angiographic catheters are being developed to allow the direct placement of the LV lead through tortuous or sharply angulated cardiac veins.

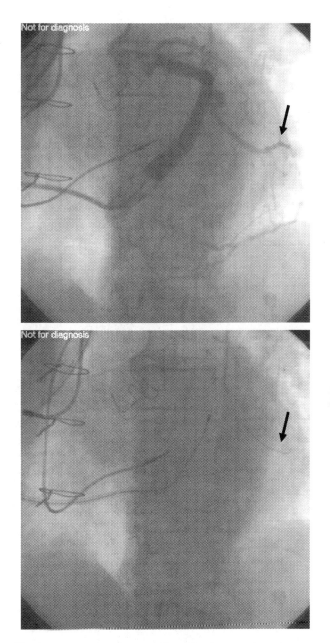

Fig. 19 Difficult access to the target cardiac vein, due to tortuosity.

20 How to manage diminutive target coronary sinus tributaries

CS tributaries may be so small as to be nearly invisible on venographic examination (Fig. 20a). Instead, angioplasty guide wires may be used to probe potential target cardiac veins, while verifying the preferred location of the vessel by fluoroscopic monitoring in the AP and 40° LAO projections (Fig. 20b,c). An over-the-wire technique is then used to advance the LV lead to its target position, confirmed in the 40° LAO fluoroscopic projection (Fig. 20d,e). This approach is also a valuable alternative to minimize the use of angiographic contrast material when implanting a CRT system in patients with renal insufficiency.

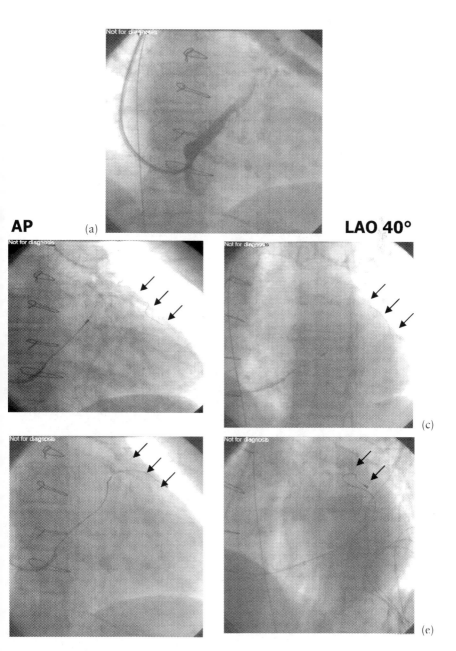

AP   (a)   **LAO 40°**

(c)

(e)

Fig. 20 Angioplasty wire used to find the LV lead route.

21 What to do when valves are in the way

Valves are commonly present in the main CS, though may not be recognized on venography. Despite the apparent ease of CS catheterization, a valve may prevent the advancement of the guiding sheath (and LV lead) toward the target vessel. Figure 21(a) illustrates the upstream occlusion of the CS, as a valve was inadvertently closed by inflation of a venography balloon catheter in the mid-CS. Resolution of this undesirable event requires withdrawal of the balloon toward the CS ostium, instead of its distal advancement. Figure 21(b) shows a second occlusive venography after more proximal re-inflation of the balloon catheter, allowing proper opacification of the entire CS and of two large tributaries.

Figures 21(c,d) are endovenous echographic images of a valve in the mid-CS which was not visible on venography (Fig. 21e). Since the valve could not be crossed, the LV lead was ultimately placed in a posterior CS tributary, after fluoroscopic confirmation of its proper position in the 40° LAO projection (Fig. 21f,g).

Figures 21(h–j) show the presence of a proximal valve near the entrance of a posterior venous tributary. A guiding sheath was placed at the CS ostium to allow the advancement of an angioplasty guide wire into the posterior venous system, and, ultimately, into a small postero-lateral vein (*). The LV lead was advanced over the wire to its final position.

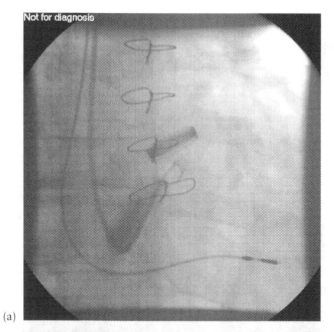

(a)

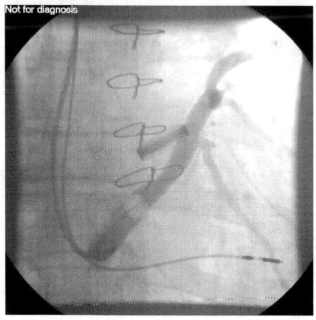

(b)

Fig. 21 (a–b) Valve located at mid CS. (*Continued.*)

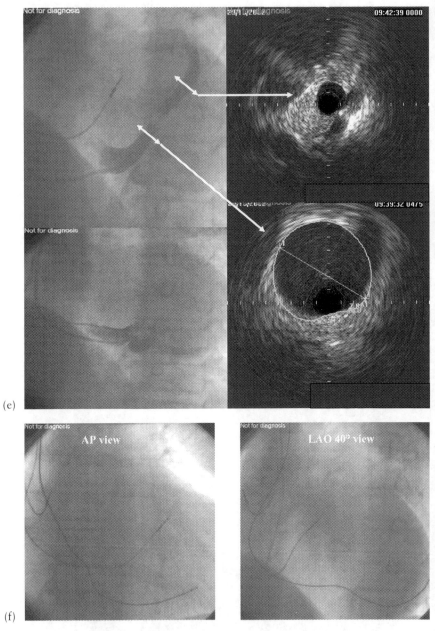

(e)

(f)

Fig. 21 (Continued.) (c–g) Valve located at mid CS.

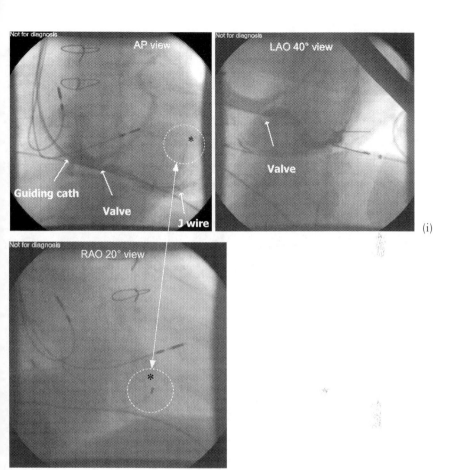

(i)

Fig. 21 (Continued.) (h–j) Valve located at the entrance of posterior vein.

22 How to implant a CRT system in the presence of a left superior vena cava

A persistent left superior vena cava is identified by direct venography or indirectly by the late opacification phase of a coronary arteriogram.

Figure 22(a) shows the introducer guide wire passing from the subclavian vein via a persistent left superior vena cava. It was decided to attempt implant of the LV lead from a right-sided approach. An angiographic balloon catheter was passed through a guiding catheter from the 'R' SVC and into the LSVC to delineate the LSVC (Fig. 22b,c).

Note that no branch vessels from the coronary sinus can be delineated because of brisk venous blood flow through the LSVC and the inability of the balloon catheter to adequately occlude the coronary sinus. A coronary arteriogram was performed to locate a cardiac vein (arrows) during levophase for lead placement (Fig. 22d,e). Successful implantation of the LV lead in the middle cardiac vein via a persistent left superior vena cava is seen in Fig. 22(f,g).

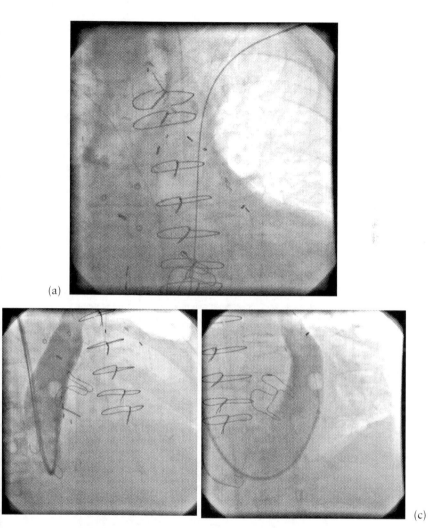

(a)

(c)

Fig. 22 (a) Guide wire in L SVC. (b,c) Persistent left superior vena cava venogram – (b) RAO, (c) LAO. (*Continued.*)

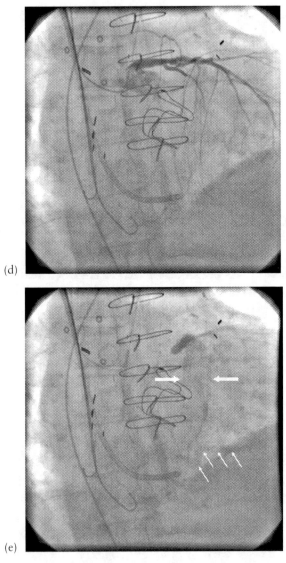

(d)

(e)

Fig. 22 (Continued.) (d,e) Angiogram to identify venous branches – (d) coronary arteriogram, (e) levophase of angiogram, coronary sinus at bold arrows, posterior-lateral cardiac vein at narrow arrows.

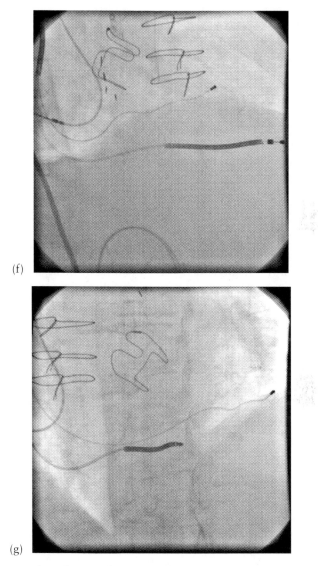

(f)

(g)

Fig. 22 (Continued.) Left SVC – final result: (f) RAO; (g) LAO.

23 Dilatation of the target cardiac vein by angioplasty techniques

Proper positioning of the LV lead may be hampered by segmental narrowing of the target cardiac vein (muscular bridging?), or by general vascular thinness. In carefully selected cases, local dilatation of the cardiac vein by conventional angioplasty techniques may be achieved to facilitate the optimal placement of the LV lead (Fig. 23a,b). After successful dilatation, the final venogram confirms a widely patent target vein now suitable for LV stimulation (Fig. 23c,d).

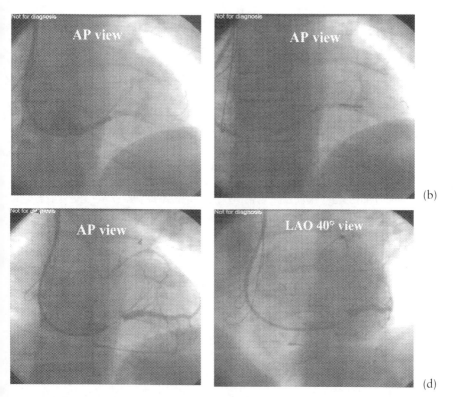

(b)

(d)

Fig. 23 Dilatation of the cardiac vein by angioplasty techniques for LV lead placement.

24 Stenting for recurrent dislodgment of the left ventricular lead

Recurrent LV lead dislodgment may be due to an inordinately wide venous system and mismatch of the lead/vessel sizes. This complication can be remedied by expanding an endovascular stent, bolstering the LV lead against the venous wall. This procedure should be reserved for cases refractory to standard techniques, since it may hamper the subsequent removal of the LV lead, should it become necessary. Figure 24(a) illustrates the placement of a stent within a posterior vein to maintain a LV lead in proper position (arrows), after the dislodgment of a previously implanted lead (*). Figure 24(b) shows the LV lead immobilized between the expanded stent and the vessel wall in a cardiac transplantation candidate.

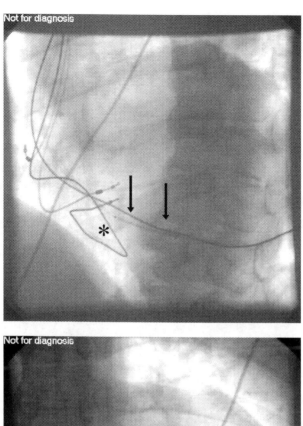

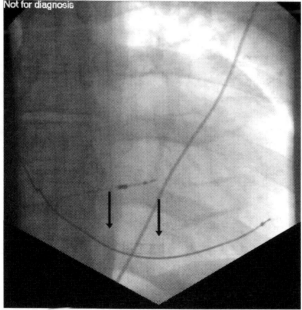

Fig. 24 Stenting for recurrent dislodgment of the left ventricular lead. This approach is not recommended as routine.

25 Assessment of the electrical signal sensed by the left ventricular lead

The recording of the LV electrogram, the peak amplitude of which coincides with the terminal portion of the surface QRS or later (Fig. 25), is one among several indicators of a properly chosen implantation site. Whether it is best measured during spontaneous rhythm versus RV pacing remains to be determined. This simple method, limited by the absence of a clear correlation between electrical and mechanical dyssynchrony, allows the exclusion of an undesirable position of the lead in the great or mid-cardiac vein.

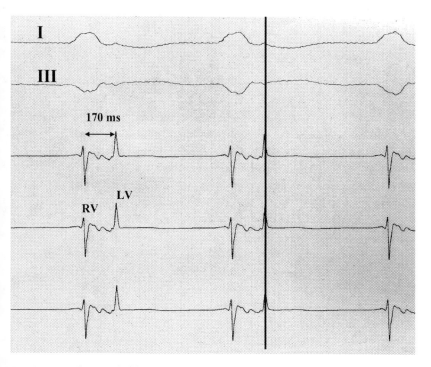

Fig. 25 Signals recorded from RV and LV leads.

26 How to avoid stimulating the left phrenic nerve

An optimal LV lead placement from hemodynamic and electrical stand-points may be defeated by the occurrence of phrenic nerve stimulation. Fine tuning of an intermediate stimulus output between LV and phrenic nerve capture is unlikely to eliminate this intolerable adverse effect, and may, on the long term, force a re-intervention to reposition the LV lead. Instead, when identified, it should prompt a search for an alternate position within the same or neighboring cardiac vein, even at the cost of less optimal electrical measurements. Figures 26(a–d) illustrate the change in LV lead position made in response to phrenic nerve stimulation observed over a long segment of a postero-lateral vein (arrows Fig. 26b) during initial CRT system implantation. Repositioning of the lead in an adjacent vein (*, Fig. 26c,d) successfully eliminated phrenic nerve stimulation, while LV capture threshold was modestly increased. A similar example is shown in Fig. 26(e,f), in a patient whose LV lead needed to be repositioned at 6 months of follow-up.

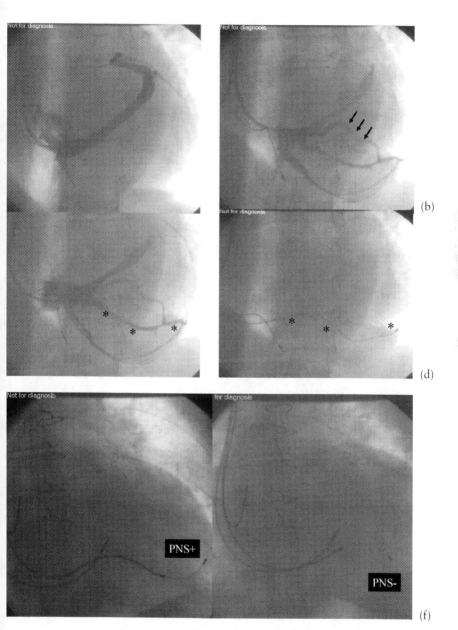

(b)

(d)

(f)

Fig. 26 LV lead repositioning due to phrenic nerve stimulation (PNS).

27 Dye extravasation and venous perforation or dissection

Dye extravasation may occur in up to 20% of cases, due to contrast material leaking from a cardiac vein and diffusing into either the pericardium or the myocardium (Fig. 27a). This may cause a persistent contrast image for 24–48 hours without clinical consequences. Frank perforation of a CS tributary has become a rare complication with the use of newer guiding instrumentation and over-the-wire leads. Perforation and/or dissection of the CS itself may result from either trauma caused by the guiding sheath or by the inflation of an oversized balloon catheter. Figure 27(b) is a radiographic image of a mid-CS dissection by a balloon catheter with abundant dye extravasation. This was associated with no circulatory consequences, and the implant procedure was uninterrupted. Figure 27(c) shows a dissection of the CS in its entire length, caused by a venous intimal tear aggravated by balloon inflation. Development of hypotension forced the discontinuation of the procedure, which was postponed for 3 weeks.

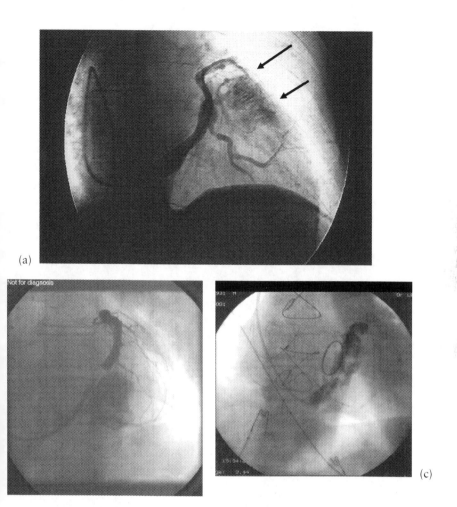

Fig. 27 (a) Dye extravasation during CS angiography: a common finding. (b,c) coronary sinus perforation/dissection.

28 How to avoid a cardiac vein dissection by the balloon catheter

Dissection within a CS tributary may also complicate the inflation of a balloon catheter, particularly when inappropriately engaged into a vein of insufficient dimensions (Fig. 28a–c). In this example, the procedure was successfully completed with the LV lead placed in an appropriate target location (Fig. 28d). This complication may be avoided by the injection of a small amount of contrast material immediately before inflating the balloon to confirm that the balloon is not engaged into the vein, and has remained within the CS lumen.

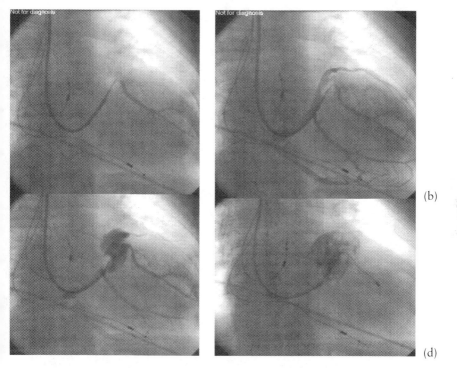

(b)

(d)

Fig. 28 Cardiac vein dissection due to inappropriate inflation of the balloon catheter.

29 How to remove the guiding sheath using the slitting technique

The guiding sheath is removed by an incision over its entire length (Fig. 29). A special cutting instrument (slitter) is adapted to the LV lead body size, and held in position strictly parallel to the long axis of the guiding sheath. While holding the slitter with one hand, the sheath is withdrawn over the blade with the other hand in a single, uninterrupted motion, without fluoroscopic monitoring. A new metallic slitter is now available, that can facilitate this particular procedure.

- **Do stabilize hand and pull catheter**
- **Do keep barrel of slitter parallel with catheter**
- **Do turn your body away from patient, pull in a single, smooth motion**

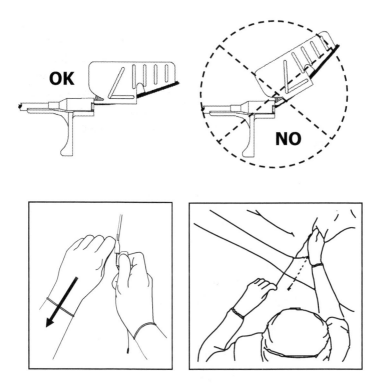

Fig. 29 Remove implant tools – slitting the guiding catheter.

30 Radiographic appearance of the final lead position of the CRT system

The proper lead placement of the CRT system should be verified in several fluoroscopic projections, including AP and 40° LAO. Figure 30(a–c) shows the placement of a triple lead system in its final position. Note the location of the LV lead body resting against the right atrial free wall and its distal tip advanced toward the LV free wall. The RV lead has been properly implanted in the mid-portion of the interventricular septum. Figure 30(d) is an example of potentially unstable LV lead placement, manifest as a loop (arrows) formed near the CS ostium (Fig. 30e).

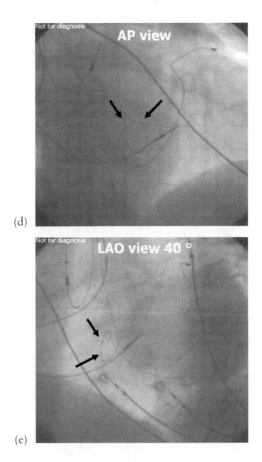

(d)

(e)

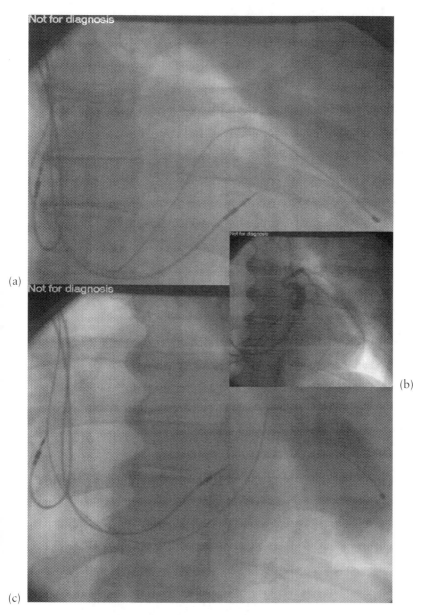

(a)

(b)

(c)

Fig. 30 (a–c) FInal lead position of the LRT system. (d,e) (opposite page) Unstable final LV lead placement.

31 How to implant a CRT device in patients with chronic atrial fibrillation

The MUSTIC AF study[4] has confirmed the therapeutic benefits of CRT in patients with chronic AF. The lead system is limited to two ventricular leads, respectively implanted in the RV and a CS tributary (Fig. 31), as described previously. Meticulous attention needs to be paid to the variations in ventricular rate observed prior to the CRT system implantation. In order to achieve reliable resynchronization, the spontaneous ventricular rate needs to be completely overdriven, and the ventricles 100% stimulated. This may, in selected patients, require ablation of the atrioventricular junction.

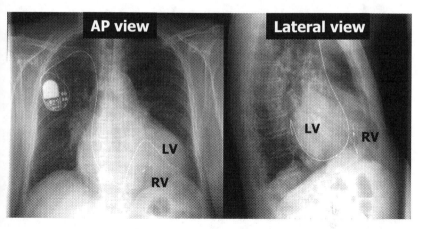

Fig. 31 AP and profile views, showing lead placement during biventricular pacing in a patient with chronic AF. Note the positions of the RV lead close to the interventricular septum and of the LV lead close to the LV lateral wall.

32 Upgrading DDD pacing to CRT

Studies are in progress to confirm the merits of upgrading a conventional DDD to an atrio-biventricular stimulation system. However, uncontrolled studies strongly suggest that an equivalent therapeutic benefit is obtainable in patients with indications for conventional single or dual chamber pacing. The patency of the subclavian vein used for implantation of the preexistent lead(s) system should be verified before insertion of the LV lead. Under fluoroscopic control, CS venography is first performed (Fig. 32a,b) and the LV lead is implanted into a target cardiac vein, as described earlier (Fig. 32c,d). A preexistent functional RV lead can be left in its original position, to eliminate risks of complications associated with its repositioning, even if not attached at an optimal site from the standpoint of ventricular resynchronization. Similar recommendations apply to an upgrade of an ICD to a CRT-ICD system.

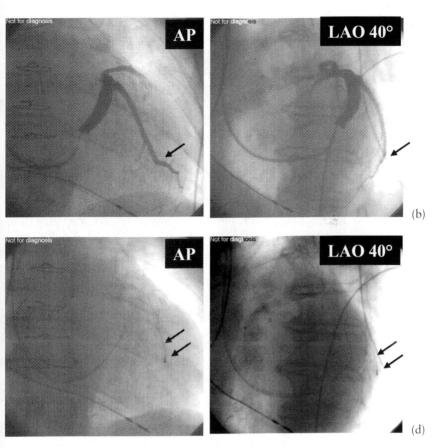

(b)

(d)

Fig. 32 LV lead implantation to upgrade DDD pacing to CRT.

33 Upgrading a CRT to a CRT-ICD system

Recipients of a CRT system may later become candidates for the addition of ICD therapy. An RV defibrillation lead should be implanted from the ipsilateral side of the previously implanted CRT leads, whether right or left, to replace the functions of the preexistent RV lead. Its placement will be determined by an optimal balance between its uses as a defibrillation versus a resynchronization lead. The choice of an active-fixation lead is preferred to allow a choice among several sites along the septum (RV, Fig. 33).

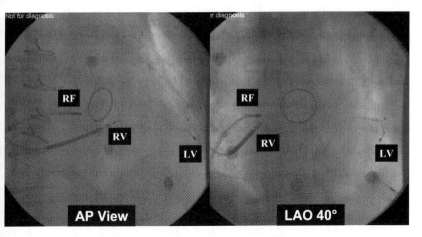

Fig. 33 Radio frequency (RF) ablation of the AV junction in a patient with chronic atrial fibrillation (AF) implanted with a biventricular CRT-ICD system. Note the vicinity between distal tips, especially of the ablation catheter (RF) and the defibrillation lead (RV).

34 Repositioning of a dislodged left ventricular lead

A dislodged LV lead should be left in place until placement of a guiding sheath into the CS and performance of a venogram (Fig. 34a,b). Prevention of recurrent lead dislodgment may require the choice of either a new target vein or a different LV lead model (Fig. 34c – Medtronic Model 4193 vs. 2187). The dislodged LV lead is removed at the very completion of the procedure.

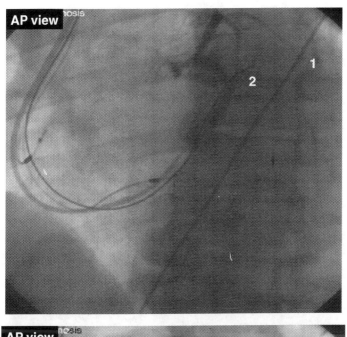

(a)

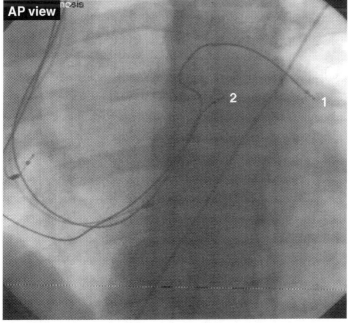

(b)

Fig. 34 LV lead repositioning in another cardiac vein (1) than the one previously selected (2). (*Continued.*)

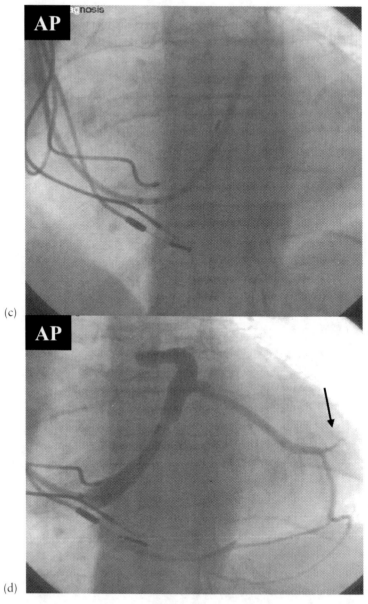

Fig. 34 (Continued.) (c) LV lead repositioning by selecting a new LV lead design. (d) CS venography.

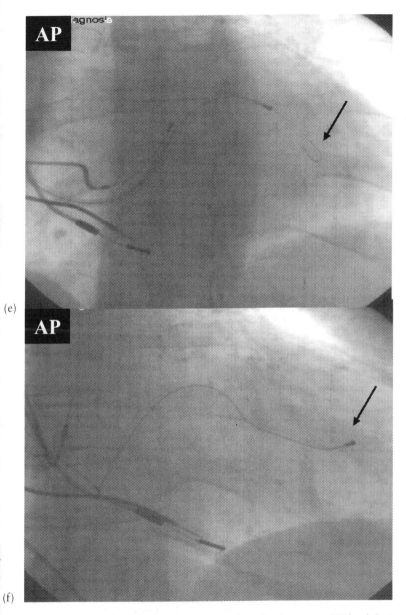

(e)

(f)

Fig. 34 (Continued.) (e) LV lead repositioning by selecting a new LV lead design. (f) Over-the-wire lead placement.

35 How to implant a four-chamber CRT system

The presence of advanced interatrial conduction block may mandate the implantation of a four-chamber CRT system, capable not only of performing standard ventricular resynchronization, but also of correcting atrial dyssynchrony. In practice, this option requires, at the end of the procedure, the implantation of an LA pacing lead (LA, Fig. 35), in addition to the previously described atrio-biventricular system. This can be accomplished with a dedicated, Medtronic Model 2188, distally curved bipolar lead placed in the proximal or mid-CS, depending on the balance between lead stability and quality of the capture threshold. The sensing performance of this LA lead is of minor importance as long as the amplitude of the right atrial electrogram is high enough. If a stable position cannot be reached, it has been recommended to implant an active fixation lead near the CS ostium, avoiding with great care attachment of the lead at the free wall level, which may cause a pericardial effusion. Though it may be tempting from a hemodynamic perspective, this configuration must be reserved to special cases since there is currently no pulse generator manufactured for true four-chamber stimulation purposes. Therefore, it forces the use of a composite atrial lead with a Y adapter, associated with a risk of oversensing at the atrial level, and interference with CRT.

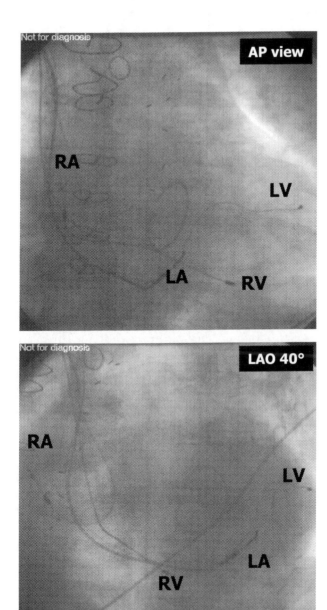

Fig. 35 Four-chamber CRT system providing atrial resynchronization between right and left atrial leads (RA and LA), together with ventricular resynchronization between right and left ventricular leads (RV and LV). This pacing configuration is not recommended as routine.

36 How to implant a biventricular, double-left ventricular lead CRT system

A new stimulation configuration, including one right and two left ventricular leads with a view to further enhance the quality of CRT, is currently being studied. After implantation of the RV lead, as described earlier, one guiding sheath is introduced into the CS to obtain a venogram and to verify that two cardiac veins are present at a sufficient distance from each other, both suitable for an over-the-wire implantation of a LV lead (great cardiac and posterior veins, Fig. 36a–d, or anterolateral and posterior veins, Fig. 36e,f). The first LV lead is implanted in the vein promising the highest stability. Another guiding sheath is then introduced into the CS to implant the second LV lead in the alternate cardiac vein. This may be a delicate procedure, at the time of leads implantation as well as when the guiding sheaths are being withdrawn (arrows in Fig. 36e), the latter starting with the sheath containing the most stable of the two leads. In both illustrative examples chosen from patients presenting with AF and complete AV block (Fig. 36a–d and Fig. 36e,f), one of the LV leads was connected to the atrial channel of a triple chamber pulse generator, programmed in DDIR mode with the shortest available AV delay.

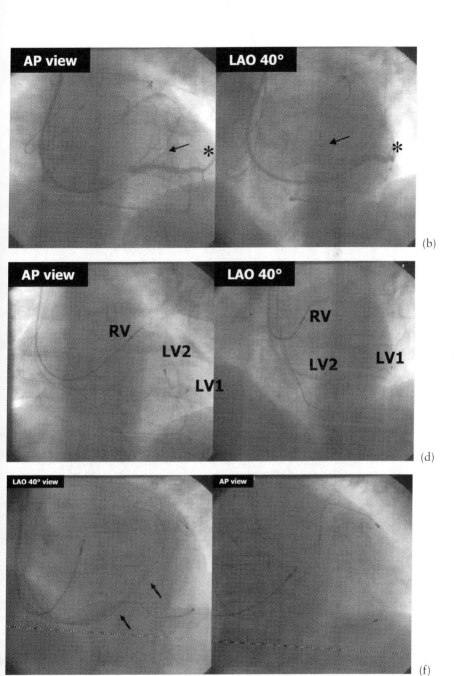

(b)

(d)

(f)

Fig. 36 Implantation of a biventricular, double left ventricular lead (LV1 and LV2) CRT system.

37 Alternatives in left ventricular lead implant failures

After failure of implantation to the LV lead, a strategy may be adopted which, in a first step, consists in implanting a triple chamber pulse generator after having joined RA and RV leads together and sealed the LV channel. In a second step, 3–4 weeks later, a choice can be made to:

1 make another attempt to catheterize a cardiac vein from an ipsi- or contralateral approach with subcutaneous lead tunnelization, while being better prepared to manage previously encountered technical obstacles, or

2 proceed directly with the implantation of an epicardial lead via thoracotomy (Fig. 37a) or, preferably, thoracoscopy (Fig. 37b) with dedicated instrumentation allowing the least invasive procedure possible.

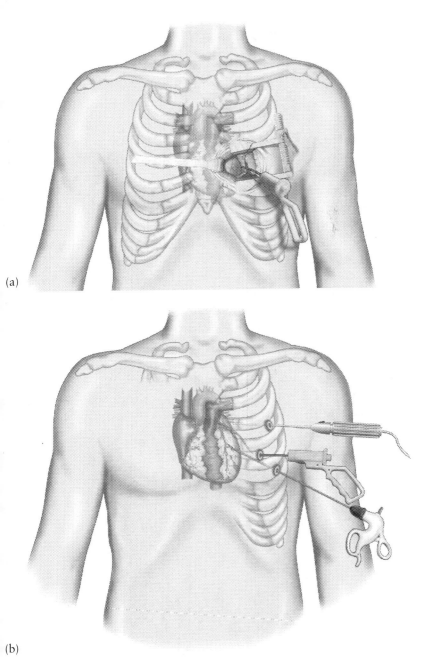

(a)

(b)

Fig. 37 (a) Lateral mini thoracotomy. (b) Thoracoscopic approach: epicardial LV implant tool.

38 Left ventricular lead extraction

The experience gathered thus far with the extraction of LV leads is limited because (a) CRT began less than 10 years ago and was validated in controlled studies only recently, with short follow-up periods during which lead extractions have been necessary, and (b) the limited life expectancy of current candidates for CRT lowers the likelihood of potential long-term LV leads dysfunction. From experimental observations, and a few dozens of cases reported at recent scientific meetings, the extraction of an LV lead implanted in a cardiac vein is usually uncomplicated. This may be due, at least partially, to the formation of less entrapping fibrosis around a lead placed in a vein, constantly exposed to circulating blood, as opposed to a lead wedged inside the trabeculated RA or RV apex.

To extract an LV lead, it is recommended to advance a stylet of suitable length to its end and apply gentle, though gradually increasing, traction (Fig. 38a) to liberate its distal extremity. The lead to be explanted is kept inside the CS to help guiding the implantation of the new lead, and is completely removed at the very end of the procedure (Fig. 38b–e). The use of instruments regularly employed to extract RV or RA leads is discouraged, particularly rigid sheaths to dissect fibrotic tissue entrapping the lead body. Likewise, traction–countertraction maneuvers should not be made, as they are the source of CS wall tears, pericardial effusion, and tamponade.

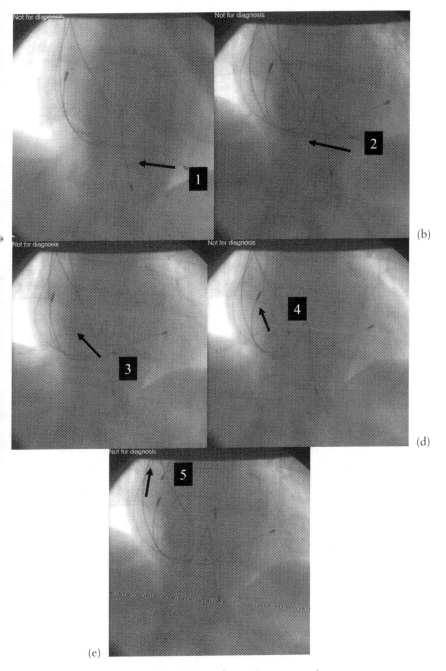

(b)

(d)

(e)

Fig. 38 LV lead extraction achieved by gentle continuous traction.

39 *Management of ventricular double counting in CRT*

Ventricular double counting is a potential complication limited to the first generation of triple chamber devices, which do not include three separate output channels. The sensing of single ventricular extrasystoles as two separate signals originating from the RV and LV, respectively, causes it. This may cause the second ventricular signal to reset and delay the post-ventricular atrial refractory period (PVARP) up to the next P wave, which falls in the refractory period and fails to initiate the next AV delay (Fig. 39). This 'self-inhibition' of CRT can be prevented by programming a PVARP < 280 ms, and by turning off the post-extrasystolic PVARP prolongation function.

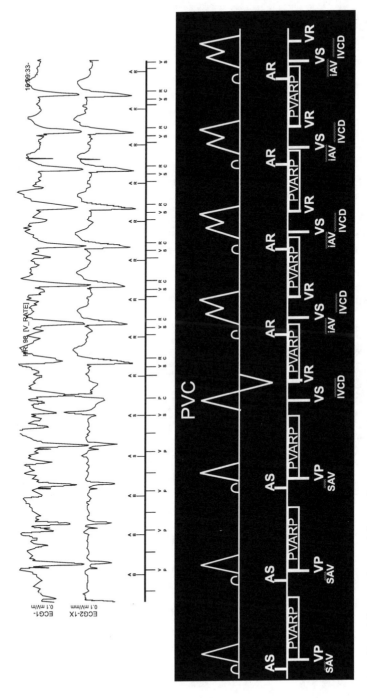

Fig. 39 Inhibition of CRT delivery due to ventricular double counting in a first-generation triple-chamber device.

40 Management of non-responders to CRT

The management of patients who do not respond to CRT should include a checklist (Fig. 40a) to address a series of questions.

1 Are the selection criteria indeed present, and is cardiac dyssynchrony confirmed echocardiographically? Does the patient suffer from evolving coronary artery disease, which may be revascularized, or from severe, irreversible LV dysfunction accounting for the refractoriness of symptoms?

2 Have the leads been properly implanted? Has the LV lead been incorrectly placed in the great cardiac vein? Does the RV apical lead cause additional uncorrected ventricular dyssynchrony? Does the RA lead properly sense atrial activity?

3 Is the AV delay optimal? In particular, in presence of a marked inter-atrial conduction delay, has the LV filling pattern remained abnormal?

4 Might ventricular resynchronization be improved by optimizing the V–V delay, which, theoretically, could contribute to an additional increase in LVEF, and further improvements in segmental contraction (Fig. 40b)?

5 Is there ventricular double counting?

6 Are there episodes of device-induced tachycardias, or spontaneous ventricular or atrial arrhythmias, which, in this context, are particularly poorly tolerated from not only rapid and irregular cardiac activity, but also from immediate loss of resynchronization? In case of recurrent paroxysmal atrial tachyarrhythmias, treatment often needs to be completed by ablation of the AV junction.

- Patient selection: Inappropriate
- Lead positioning: LV, RV, RA
- AV delay tuning
- VV delay tuning
- CRT delivery: Inappropriate PM functioning
- Arrhythmias: Pacemaker mediated or spontaneous

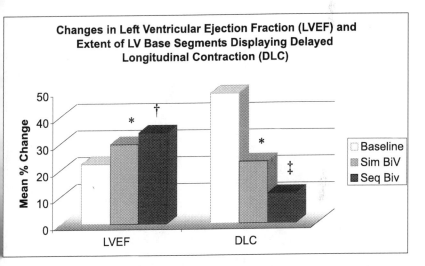

Fig. 40 (a) What to check in non-responders. (b) Sequential (Seq) vs. simultaneous (Sim) biventricular resynchronization (BiV) for Severe Heart Failure. * P < 0.01 vs. baseline, † P < 0.01 Seq vs. Sim, ‡ P < 0.05 Seq vs. Sim.[27]

References

1   Grines CL, Bashore TM, Boudoulas H, Olson S, Shafer P, and Wooley CF. Functional abnormalities in isolated left bundle branch block. The effect of interventricular asynchrony. *Circulation* 1989; **79**: 845–53.

2   Bradley DJ, Bradley EA, Baughman KL, *et al.* Cardiac resynchronization and death from progressive heart failure: a meta-analysis of randomized controlled trials. *J Am Med Assoc* 2003; **289**: 730–40.

3   www.uchsc.edu/cvi/HFSA%20V3%20Late%20Breaker-presented%209.24.03.pdf

4   Cleland JGF, Daubert JC, Erdmann E, *et al.*, on behalf of The CARE-HF study Steering Committee and Investigators. The CARE-HF study (CArdiac REsynchronisation in Heart Failure study): rationale, design and end-points. *Eur J Heart Fail* 2001; **3**: 481–9.

5   Leclercq C, Cazeau S, Ritter P, *et al.* A pilot experience with permanent biventricular pacing to treat advanced heart failure. *Amer Heart J* 2000; **140**(6): 862–70.

6   Gras D, Leclercq C, Tang A, *et al.* Cardiac resynchronization therapy in advanced heart failure the multicenter InSync clinical study. *Eur J Heart Fail* 2002; **4**: 311–20.

7   Chan KL, Tang ASL, Achilli A, *et al.* Functional and echocardiographic improvement following multisite biventricular pacing for congestive heart failure. *Can J Cardiol* 2003; **19**(4): 387–90.

8   Kühlkamp V. Initial experience with an implantable cardioverter-defibrillator incorporating cardiac resynchronizatoion therapy. *J Am Coll Cardiol* 2002; **39**: 790–7.

9   Cazeau S, Leclercq C, Lavergne T, *et al.*, for the Multisite Stimulation In Cardiomyopathies (MUSTIC) Study Investigators. Effects of multisite biventricular pacing in patients with heart failure and intraventricular conduction delay. *N Engl J Med* 2001; **344**: 873–80.

10 Duncan A, Wait D, Gibson D, and Daubert JC. Left ventricular remodeling and haemodynamic effects of multisite biventricular pacing in patients with left ventricular systolic dysfunction and activation disturbances in sinus rhythm: substudy of the MUSTIC (Multisite Stimulation in Cardiomyopathies) trial. *Eur Heart J* 2003; **24**: 430–41.

11 Stellbrink C, Breithardt O, Franke A, *et al.* Impact of cardiac resynchronization therapy using hemodynamically optimized pacing on left ventricular remodeling in patients with congestive heart failure and ventricular conduction disturbances. *J Am Coll Cardiol* 2001; **38**: 1957–65.

12 Auricchio A, Stellbrink C, Sack S, *et al.* Long-term clinical effect of hemodynamically optimized cardiac resynchronization therapy in patients with heart failure and ventricular conduction delay. *J Am Coll Cardiol* 2002; **39**: 1895–8.

13 Leclercq C, Walker S, Linde C, *et al.* Comparative effects of permanent biventricular and right-univentricular pacing in heart failure patients with chronic atrial fibrillation. *Eur Heart J* 2002; **23**: 1780–7.

14 Abraham WT, Fisher WG, Smith AL, *et al.* Cardiac resynchronization in chronic heart failure. *N Engl J Med* 2002; **346**: 1845–53.

15 St. John Sutton MG, Plappert T, Abraham WT, *et al.* Effect of cardiac resynchronization on left ventricular size and function in chronic heart failure. *Circulation* 2003; **107**: 1985–90.

16 Auricchio A, Stellbrink C, Butter C, *et al.* Clinical efficacy of cardiac resynchronization therapy using left ventricular pacing in heart failure patients stratified by severity of ventricular conduction delay. *J Am Coll Cardiol* 2003; **42**: 2109–16.

17 Young JB, Abraham WT, Smith AL, *et al.* Combined cardiac resynchronization and implantable cardioverter defibrillation in advanced chronic heart failure. *J Am Med Assoc* 2003; **289**: 2685–94.

18 Higgins SL, Hummel JD, Niazi IK, *et al.* Cardiac resynchronization therapy for the treatment of heart failure in patients with intraventricular conduction delay and malignant ventricular tachyarrhythmias. *J Am Coll Cardiol*, 2003; **42**: 1454–9.

19 Young JB, Abraham WT. Cardiac resynchronization limits disease progression in patients with mild heart failure and an indication for an ICD – results of a randomized study. *Circulation* 2003 [AHA abstract] .

20 Bristow MR, *et al.* HFSA 2003 Presentation accessed at www.uchsc.edu/cvi on September 30, 2003.

21 Søgaard P, Egelblad H, Kim WY, Jensen HK, Pedersen AK, Kristensen BØ, and Mortensen PT. Tissue Doppler imaging predicts improved systolic performance and reversed left ventricular remodeling during long-term cardiac resynchronization therapy. *J Am Coll Cardiol* 2002; **40**(4): 723–30.

22 Nelson GS, Berger RD, Fetics BJ, *et al.* Left ventricular or biventricular pacing improves cardiac function at diminished energy cost in patients with dilated cardiomyopathy and left bundle-branch block. *Circulation* 2000; **102**: 3053–9.

23 Abraham WT, on behalf of the Multicenter InSync Randomized Clinical Evaluation (MIRACLE) Investigators and Coordinators. Rationale and design of a randomized clinical trial to assess the safety and efficacy of cardiac resynchronization therapy in patients with advanced heart failure: The Multicenter InSync Randomized Clinical Evaluation (MIRACLE). *J Cardiac Failure* 2000; **6**(4): 369–80.

24 Greenberg JM, *et al.*, Safety of implantation of cardiac resynchronization devices: a review of major biventricular pacing trials. *Pacing Clin Electrophysiol* 2003; **26**(4) [abstract 93].

25 Daubert J, *et al.* Long term stability of a left ventricular over the wire pacing lead. *Pacing Clin Electrophysiol* 2003; **26**(4) [abstract 329].

26 Leclercq C, Walker S, Linde C, Clementy J, Marshall AJ, Ritter P, Djiane P, Mabol P, Levy T, Gadler F, Bailleul C, and Daubert JC, on behalf of the MUSTIC study group. Comparative effects of permanent biventricular and right-univentricular pacing in heart failure patients with chronic atrial fibrillation. *Eur Heart J* 2002; **23**: 1780–7.

27 Sogaard P, Egeblad H, Pedersen AK, Kim WY, Kristensen BO, Hansen PS, and Mortensen PT. Sequential versus simultaneous biventricular resynchronization for severe heart failure: evaluation by tissue Doppler imaging. *Circulation* 2002; **106**: 2078–84.

Index

angiography
  coronary sinus 2, 3, 26
  see also venograms
angioplasty, dilatation of target cardiac
    veins 56–7
atrial dyssynchrony, four-chamber CRT
    system in correction of 82–3
atrial fibrillation (AF)
  chronic, patients with 72–3, 77
  paroxysmal 22
atrio-ventricular (AV) block 2

biventricular double-left ventricular lead
    CRT system 84–5
biventricular (BIV) pacing 73
  trials 25

cannulation, *see* catheterization/
    cannulation
cardiac dyssynchrony, *see* atrial
    dyssynchrony; ventricular
    dyssynchrony
cardiac resynchronization therapy, *see*
    CRT
cardiac vein
  choice of, for LV lead placement 2
  dilatation of target vein 56–7
  dissection, avoidance of 66–7
  dye extravasation 64–5
  lateral, venogram not showing 40–41
CARE-HF trial 6, 8
catheterization/cannulation, coronary
    sinus 32–5, 36–7
catheters 16, 17
checklists
  non-responders 92–3
  preimplantation 16–17
COMPANION trial 6, 7
complications of CRT 1, 2
Contak CD trial 7, 25
coronary sinus (CS)
  angiography 2, 3, 26
  catheterization/cannulation 32–5,
    36–7
  complex anatomy 44–5
  LV lead placement 2

myocardial bridge over 38–9
  perforation/dissection of 64–5
  valves obstructing advancement of
    guiding sheath 26, 48–51
  venogram, before left ventricular lead
    placement 26–9
  venous anatomy 26–9
coronary sinus ostium
  avoiding dissection of 36–7
  catheterization/cannulation 32, 35
  displacement of 32
coronary sinus tributaries
  diminutive 46
  pacing left ventricle via 24–5
  perforation of 64–5
CRT (cardiac resynchronization
    therapy)
  background ix, 1
  clinical benefits 6–7
  complications 1, 2
  efficacy of 7
  impact on survival 6
  implantation 3
  mechanisms of improvement during
    12–13
  non-responders, management
    checklist 92–3
  situations of doubtful therapeutic
    value 14
  studies 6–7
  see also pacing
CRT systems
  biventricular double-left ventricular
    lead 84–5
  four-chamber system 82–3
  upgrading from DDD system 74–5
  upgrading to CRT-ICD system 76–7
CRT-ICD system
  upgrade of CRT system to 76–7
  upgrade of ICD system to 74–5

DDD pacing, upgrading to CRT 74–5
dilated cardiomyopathy (DCM) 5, 8, 9
Doppler echocardiography
  evaluation of atrial electromechanical
    delays 23

identifying ventricular dyssynchrony
    10–11
dye extravasation 64–5
dyssynchrony, *see* atrial dyssynchrony;
    ventricular dyssynchrony

echocardiography
    evaluation of atrial electromechanical
        delays 23
    identifying ventricular dyssynchrony
        10–11
Eustachian valve 32

French Pilot trial 7

guiding sheath, slitting technique for
    removal of 68–9

heart failure management ix
heart rate, variability 12
hemodynamic function, ventricular
    dyssynchrony altering 4–5

ICD (implantable cardioverter
    defibrillator) system, upgrading
    to CRT-ICD system 74–5
inotropic drugs 12, 13
instrumentation 3
    preimplantation checklist 16–17
InSync trial 7
InSync ICD trial 7
InSync III trial 25

lateral cardiac vein, venogram not
    showing 40–41
lead placement
    final position, radiographic
        appearance 70–71
    see also left ventricular lead
        placement
left bundle branch block (LBBB) 2
left phrenic nerve stimulation 2–3
    avoiding 62–3
left superior vena cava 52–5
left ventricle
    high pacing thresholds 42–3
    pacing sites 31
    pacing via coronary sinus tributary
        24–5
    remodeling, reversal of 12, 13

systolic function improvement 12, 13
left ventricular ejection fraction (LVEF)
    4, 5, 6, 12
left ventricular (LV) lead
    assessment of electrical signal sensed
        by 60
    biventricular double-left ventricular
        lead CRT system 84–5
    extraction 88–9
    implant failures, alternatives 86–7
    repositioning after dislodgement
        78–81
    stenting for recurrent dislodgment of
        58–9
left ventricular (LV) lead placement 1–3
    choice of vein 2
    coronary sinus venogram before 26–9
    optimal positioning 30–31
    right- *v.* left-sided approach 18–19
    venogram not showing lateral cardiac
        vein 40–41
left ventricular (LV) stimulation 20, 24,
    40

MIRACLE (Multicenter InSync
    Randomized Clinical Evaluation)
    trial 7, 25
    exclusion criteria 15
MIRACLE ICD trial 7, 25
MIRACLE ICD II trial 7
mitral regurgitation, decrease in 12, 13
MUSTIC (Multisite Stimulation in
    Cardiomyopathies) study 7
    exclusion criteria 15
MUSTIC AF study 7, 72
myocardial bridges, over coronary sinus
    38–9
myocardial oxygen consumption 12, 13

neuro-hormonal activity 12

oxygen, myocardial consumption 12, 13

pacing
    biventricular 73
    left atrial 24
    left ventricular 24–5, 31, 42–3
    right atrial 22–3
    right ventricular 20–21
    trials, biventricular (BIV) 25

upgrading DDD to CRT 74–5
PATH CHF trial 7
PATH CHF II trial 7
patient selection criteria ix, 8–9
phrenic nerve stimulation, *see* left
    phrenic nerve stimulation
post-ventricular atrial refractory period
    (PVARP) 90–91

radiography, appearance of final lead
    position 70–71
renal insufficiency 46
right atrium
    pacing 22–3
    sensing 22–3
right bundle branch block (RBBB)
    trauma 1, 2, 20
right ventricular lead implantation 1, 2,
    3, 20–21
right ventricular pacing 20–21
right ventricular stimulation 20–21

stenting, for recurrent dislodgment of LV
    lead 58–9
subclavian vein
    exclusion 19
    puncture 2

survival, impact of CRT 6

tamponade 36
Thebesian valve 32, 34
thoracoscopy 86–7
thoracotomy 86–7

valves, obstructing advancement of
    guiding sheath 26, 48–51
veins, *see* cardiac vein; subclavian vein
venograms
    coronary sinus, before left ventricular
        lead placement 26–9
    to establish target veins 42–3
    with myocardial bridge 38
    not showing lateral cardiac vein
        40–41
    see also angiography
venous perforation/dissection 64–5
ventricular double counting 90–91
ventricular dyssynchrony 9
    assessment 10–11
    Doppler echocardiography
        identifying 10–11
    hemodynamic function and 4–5
    as selection criteria 8
ventricular filling 12, 13